THE 7 FUNDAMENTALS OF A
HIGHLY
SUCCESSFUL
ALLIED
HEALTH CLINIC

The first seven steps to ensuring you grow the Allied Health business of your dreams

Jason Pilgrim

Founder of the Global Kaizen Group and other industry-leading Allied Health companies

The developer and owner of Australia's most awarded Allied Health Business Blueprint

The 7 Fundamentals of a Highly Successful
Allied Health Clinic
First Published in 2015

This publication is designed to provide accurate and authoritative information in regard to the subject matters covered. It is sold with the understanding that neither the author nor the publisher is engaged in rendering legal, accounting, investment or other professional services. The author and publisher advise that if assistance in these aforementioned areas is required, then the services of a professional should be sought.

To those who love the Allied Health industry as much as I do. Although very tough at times I hope that it is as kind to you as it has been to me.

I would like to dedicate this book to the inspirational and hardworking Exercise Physiologists and Allied Health professionals who use their passion and drive to help empower their patients to achieve greater outcomes in their lives.

This book has been many years in the making with my many trials and tribulations working with dozens of Allied Health companies. I hope that everyone who reads this book will be better equipped with the key fundamentals and strategies to either start and grow their own successful Allied Health clinic or to take their existing business and grow it into the Allied Health clinic of their dreams.

Here's to *Empowering and Inspiring Lifestyle Abundance,*

Acknowledgments

If you ever see a turtle sitting on a fence post, you can be sure he didn't get there on his own.

To my loving, supportive and very patient wife, Vanessa, who does not always get the credit she deserves, I couldn't do what I do without you. To my three beautiful girls, Olivia, Georgia and Isla who always enable me to keep a smile on my face and feel grounded. To my parents and close friends that have always been so supportive of my endeavours regardless of how crazy some of them may sound and how stubborn I have been at many times. Thank you to all of you for being such a major influence in my life.

A massive thank you to the coaches and mentors who I have been aligned with, it really has been a huge privilege to know each of you and to have been fortunate enough to learn and grow from your years of experience and wisdom. Brad Sugars, Taki Moore, Dale Beaumont, Les Brown – thank you all very much.

To my fellow Jedi masters, we've all come so far and it has been an absolute honour to be a part of the journey for all of us together. I look forward to many more adventures and business dealings in the future.

A huge thank you to Leanne Smith, for always being there for myself and my family and doing her best to keep me in line. And to my amazing In2 Motion team over the years, a massive thank you. Rarely does a business owner get to work with the amazing people who I've had the privilege of doing so with and to be given the opportunity to constantly try new ideas and innovations with such great people is a truly humbling honour for me.

To my very good friend and cofounder of the Global Kaizen Group, Andrew Boyle, thank you for being a part of this journey with me. To our whole Kaizen team from Cassandra Grosso through to our fantastic virtual assistants led by the amazing Maria Lilia Gunda, thank you very much for your passion and ongoing commitment.

And finally, to all of the patients, clients and customers over many years. Thank you very much for enabling me to live out my vision each and every day. It is truly a blessing that I'm exceptionally grateful for and I can't wait to see what the future holds.

.... And also to the entrepreneurs and business leaders who have inspired me that I haven't met personally, a massive thank you. Jim Rohn, Zig Ziglar, Simon Sinek, Steve Jobs, Richard Branson, Marshall Goldsmith, Tony Hsieh, Grant Cardone and Malcolm Gladwell.

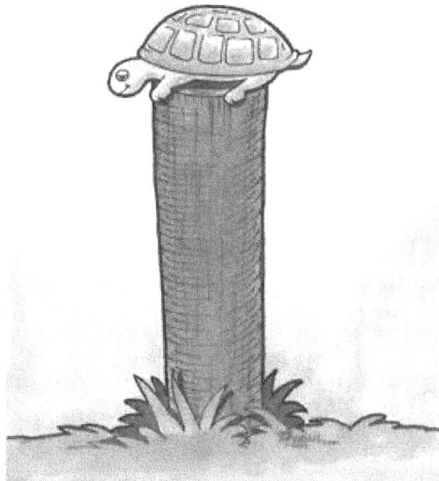

Contents

Chapter 1:

Why / Vision

Why is it that you do what you do? Why is it that you work so hard, in often very trying situations? Why do you keep going with what seems to be too many rules and regulations with loads of paperwork and red tape to be completed in order for just a simple bill <u>to be</u> paid? Well, the good news is you're not alone. There are a large number of your colleagues in the industry who feel exactly the same way.

The first step in securing clarity for the direction of your career and business within the Allied Health industry is to clearly define your *why*. I'm not talking about what you do or how you do it. More so, I'm trying to get to the very crux of *why* you do what you do each and every day. It is having this clear understanding of *why* you do what you do that is the cornerstone, and the very first step to be undertaken, on your path to future success.

We always hear of people defining who they are and all too often we read motivational pieces from people who are trying to inspire us to find ourselves and what we're really about. Unfortunately, the common fault with these pieces of literature is that they are all too generic and based around generalised principles designed to make you think in an overarching context. What I'm talking about is actually much more specific to our industry. It's about knowing who you are as a person but more so knowing and understanding exactly what it is that you're wanting to achieve within the industry as an Allied Health professional.

As Simon Sinek said for many years, "People don't buy what you do. People buy why you do it." It is for this exact reason that knowing what your purpose is and why you do things must be the first clear step forward in getting your business goals on track.

Let's look at this from our client's point of view. They quite simply have a multitude of other industry professionals that they choose instead of coming and seeing yourself and although there are other factors that will influence this decision to become a patient of yours (including services, niche, guarantees, value for money and reputation,) having a clear understanding of your own personal *why* will greatly influence the image that your business puts forward in the marketplace. Your *'why'* will be one of the key drivers in deciding the way in which you market and promote your company to the wider demographic of possible patients.

Understanding the core driver that gets you out of bed in the morning is often a challenge for many practitioners to fully understand. It is very easy for us to make a sweeping statement such as "we wanted to help people and that's why we got into the industry." Other examples include wanting to be involved within the exercise and sports field due to a previous sporting background you might have had or it may simply be that you've always been fit and healthy and wanted to work in that type of industry. Whatever it happens to be, just remember that there is no right and wrong. However, I'm encouraging you to dig deeper than simply saying a generalised statement. Look inside yourself and really analyse what it is that you stand for and what you greatly desire to see happen in your career and business above all else. It is only then that you will truly know what your *why* is.

Often a business owner will spend more time designing their business logo than defining their *why*. We must keep in mind that logos are just logos without the clarity of *why*. Logos need to have meaning and customers need to know what they stand for.

Often when we are a long way through the process of defining our personal *why*, we get overconfident and just settle for what we have decided on without investing the time into getting it perfect. The best way to test your *why* is to use a "Celery Test." Only then will you truly know whether your *why* is strong enough.

Once you have an understanding of your core reason for doing what you do, the next step in this process is using this understanding and personal alignment to formulate your business vision. I believe that this business vision is one of the key factors to ensure your Allied Health business takes off at a rapid rate and doesn't just see you treading water for the first few years of your career.

Another one of the biggest challenges I see when discussing people's visions is that most people don't often think big enough. They are often limited by underlying fears. These fears tend to be based on a concern that they may be unable to achieve their set goal, or that achieving such a high goal will leave them at a new precarious and unknown height, unsure how to sustain their growth.

For most people having the ability to dream big is something that they're not comfortable with and as a result, it is something many people don't ever spend enough time thinking about and laying the foundations for.

I believe that in many cases it is because some of the people closest to us discourage us from dreaming big. As kids we all used to dream about some amazing things we wanted to do in our lives but as we progressed into older childhood years, it was often friends, family or teachers at our school who told us not to be silly and be realistic when we told them we wanted to be an astronaut or something way out there. Why is it that we let people around us reign in our dreams and try to discourage us from doing something amazing? For me, I completely understand that not everyone can be an astronaut but I believe if that's what you really want to do, then everyone should be encouraging and supportive and help you do everything in your power to achieve such a dream.

By keeping in mind reflections on our childhood upbringings we can better understand why most of us fail to dream at a big enough level to inspire ourselves to drive harder and faster each and every day and achieve what we really want in life.

The designing of a business vision is something that is a very complex and often long process to successfully achieve. It is not a simple process of writing down a bunch of words in a sentence and saying that's your business vision because let's face it, you know yourself that you're not being true to your own vision. How do you expect other people to buy this tongue-in-cheek vision you are trying to put forward? Be true to yourself and invest the time and effort into finding your own personal *why* and then enabling yourself to extrapolate this into the long-term vision of your company and exactly what it is you're wanting to achieve.

Find clarity and detail in your vision. Look at exactly what it looks like in five and ten years' time. Maybe your vision is based around how many people your business needs to employ. Maybe it's based around how many locations or clinics you want to have working in particular communities. Maybe it's actually focused on a charity that you have a personal affiliation to such as a cancer foundation and may result in the business vision being more than just about helping patients but also serving to raise several million dollars in funds to open your own cancer treatment hospital in the local community. Regardless of what it is, I greatly encourage you to work hard with your own thoughts and with those in your team to ensure that you are able to find this common vision, one you truly believe underpins what your business is all about.

Once you truly have this clarity around your business vision, the majority of the direction for your business marketing and great strategies are focused around the promotion of your vision and what it is you, your team and your business set out to achieve. The reality is simply that clients of a new business will always buy the story of a business, one that has a clear understanding of who they are, where they're going and what it is they're wanting to achieve rather than simply buying from a company or person that has no real direction. This is not to say that you can be insincere in what you put forward but once you truly understand where your personal passion lies and your overall vision of what you and your company wants to achieve, the rest becomes quite easy to develop.

One of my companies, the Global Kaizen Group, works significantly with dozens of Allied Health companies using multiple strategies to help people find their inner drivers and the reason why they do what they do. Our next step is to then work with the business owners and in some cases their team members, to develop the team vision and enable this to be the catalyst which can drive their business forward.

Achievement comes when you reach your goal, when you obtain what you want, but success ultimately comes when you are in clear pursuit of *WHY* you want it.

Everyone has a *why*. Every company has a *why*. But the company is always a *what*. The company is a tangible thing a founder does to ultimately prove their *why*.

So Step One must be to find your personal drivers and your *why*. Have a firm understanding of why you do what you do and what gets you out of bed in the morning, Use this as the foundations for the development of your personal and business vision. This has to be the first step and unfortunately many people in the Allied Health industry, still don't really know who they are and what it is they're wanting to achieve. As a result, they find themselves floundering and not completely happy with their direction. Albeit they may be in great workplaces and have fantastic jobs and they may be achieving great things within the industry but it is not what they want to do or who they want to be. I encourage everyone to find this *why* as the first platform step to creating the business you ultimately desire.

Chapter 2:

Self-discipline and the business owner

One of the biggest challenges I see in most Allied Health practices is that many business owners are very dedicated to patient outcomes, so much so that they are prepared to personally hamper their own well-being, detract from the business moving forward or just in general, do everything for their patients at the expense of their own future longevity.

This mentality is fraught with danger and is a recipe for significant pain and suffering for the business owner.

I would greatly encourage everyone to read the book *The Slight Edge* written by Jim Olsen. It is a very easy read and it guides people through the early stages of business and adapting the self-discipline structures and habits that surround the successful start to any new business.

Ultimately, we all see ourselves as being disciplined, hard-working and dedicated. Most people reading this section of my book will probably actually feel like it is not applicable to themselves as we all have this deep-seated feeling of self-discipline towards our own application to tasks. However, if you actually look a little deeper and be true to yourself, there are very few of us who can honestly say they have this habitual routine of good self-discipline down to a fine art.

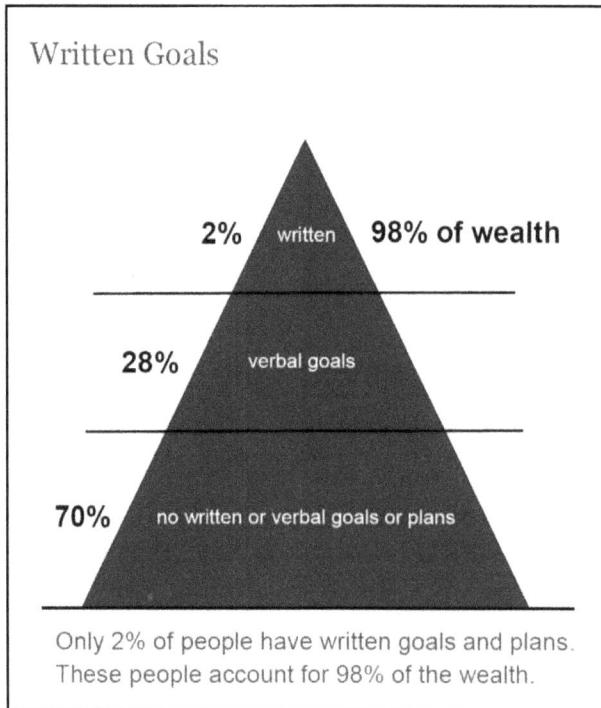

Written Goals

2% written   98% of wealth

28%   verbal goals

70%   no written or verbal goals or plans

Only 2% of people have written goals and plans. These people account for 98% of the wealth.

When we honestly look at ourselves and the role that we play within our own businesses, we all need to be truthful and admit that we allow too much procrastination to occur. In the early stages of our own business and career we often simply put off the hard decisions and fail to complete the most important and essential tasks. We consider to do them later opting to come back to them after doing a less important and less urgent task. There is no example more evident than the way we will constantly enable social media and emails to interrupt major thought processes and the completing of these more essential and urgent tasks that should have our complete and undivided attention.

Having a default diary in place for yourself is one of the simplest tasks in mastering improved effectiveness and outcomes in your business. Using a default diary to structurally add items such as manager time, owner time, exercise, meal breaks, admin time, as well as many other tasks, including sales, operations and finance is critical in establishing a set structure prior to enabling patients to be booked into your diary. Unfortunately, I see most Allied Health businesses running in the completely opposite fashion. Patients are constantly booked into their diaries and then they try to fit in the essential and very important tasks for business development and growth in and around the small snippets of spare time between patients. This is one of the worst things you can possibly do if you are wanting your business to actually grow and succeed. Operating in this way does not allow you the opportunity to immerse yourself into these important avenues for your business.

The biggest fear in these situations is based around the fact that you may be scared of losing patients because of your lack of time availability to see them. Surprisingly, it's actually the complete opposite. In most cases, and none more so highlighted in the medical and health industries, the less time you have available for appointments when portrayed to patients in the right way is actually seen by your patients as a measure of your success and the desire for so many people to want to see you and your team for the services you provide. This mentality is highlighted by the waiting lists seen for various types of specialists within the medical field.

Self-discipline also revolves around many other areas of your business. Keeping accurate business records and tracking progress and data metrics which I discussed later in this book are also key factors to ensure your business success. Often these are seen from the business owner as being boring and hence, the attention to detail is not given in these areas. In many situations it is also that the business owner doesn't actually know the benefit of this type of data and as a result, this lack of understanding of how to use it is perceived as a waste of time in collecting the data in the first place and hence, the business owner stops completing this process. The self-discipline to ensure that adequate time is allocated to these crucial areas is essential for your business success.

The keeping of fine details is a discipline that is often overlooked by business owners. One such example is the keeping of a black book with fine details about each of the key members of a medical practice is a discipline that although it takes only a small amount of time to complete and keep updated, it is often overlooked and this type of tool is one of the most beneficial ways to ensure future success and communication with each medical practice you are aligned with.

There are many aspects to self-discipline and there are quite a few tried and tested successful strategies that we guide our members through at our conferences and other business bootcamps within the Global Kaizen Group business development programs we offer. These systems and templates have foolproof measures in place to ensure guaranteed success, improved self-discipline and habits and systems ensuring greater accountability for you moving forward. Overall, you have a more effective business working at a more efficient pace and achieving greater necessary gains as a net result of these simple improvements.

Chapter 3:

Education and personal growth

Valuing ongoing continual education is something that is well-entrenched into the mindset of Allied Health professionals. We are all strongly encouraged to go to seminars, complete webinars, read journal articles and be continually striving to improve and develop our technical ability.

The limiting factor of this is that the majority, if not all of this advice, centres around us completing large amounts of technical professional growth and although this is exceptionally important, it is often not the most needed ongoing education for most business owners in the Allied Health field.

For most Allied Health professions, we see a deficit in the ongoing education related to their business acumen. Our university training prepares us for the technical and scientific aspects of our careers, but barely touches on the business training many of us require as our careers progress.

None of my comments above are a criticism but simply an observation highlighting one of the biggest challenges all of us are faced with when first stepping out into the Allied Health private practice world.

Over the years I've spent an extensive amount of money on my ongoing education with more than $250,000 on learning how to manage a successful business being spent in the last five to six years. Although this may seem like an exorbitant amount of money and yes, granted it is a very large sum of money, this has merely been a minimal investment *into* the benefit on the return on investment I have seen.

I have been a big supporter of gaining business mentors and coaches and learning from the very best who have gone before me. Early on I often had the mindset that "I'm the best one to make my own decisions." However, I have come to realise that in nearly every situation a mentor or colleague has also been faced with the exact situations I face. In many cases a mentor can easily assist and guide me past speed bumps and onto smoother roads without fuss, something I was unable to achieve myself. A support network is crucial to business and personal growth.

One thing I've learnt over the years is that personal growth and ongoing education towards achieving excellence is an endless pursuit. To grow and develop we must always appreciate the need to continually challenge ourselves. An understanding of the analogy that "If a tree isn't growing, then it's dying," reminds us to continually strive for growth and development. One aspect of ongoing education is the fact that accountability really is one of the major keys to successfully growing and developing at an exponential rate. Having mentors and buddies who are travelling the same path as yourself, who you can turn to and lean on for support and also gauge feedback regarding new strategies and/or challenges you may be experiencing, is so valuable that it's impossible to put a dollar amount on such benefit.

As one of the founders of the Global Kaizen Group, I considered the company's name carefully and used our goal in the name of our business. The business name is based off the Japanese proverb of the word *Kaizen* which literally means "continuous improvement in your personal and professional life each and every day through the elimination of waste." So much of the Global Kaizen Group is based exactly on this –continual improvement day after day, making small incremental benefits to ourselves personally and professionally. Having our business named so closely with this word and principle, is just another small way for us to put our public accountability on display and ensure that we are always living up to what we say we are aiming for.

The late great Jim Rohn is always famously quoted and one of the best things he ever said was, "Never wish life was easier. Wish that you were better." If that isn't more validation that you need to work harder on yourself each and every day to improve and get better, then I'm not sure what is.

So develop a learning plan for yourself and don't just have it revolved around the technical aspect of your skills. For those starting up their Allied Health business or in the early stages of their business growth, having a clearly defined learning plan surrounding your business development expertise and the many facets that align with this is critically important to your success. Please don't think for a minute that by reading one business accounting textbook or simply speaking with your accountant on a quarterly basis that you will have all the business guidance and learnings you need to succeed. It is a journey that involves daily, weekly and monthly commitments to ongoing learning and one of the best ways to do this is by being accountable to other like-minded Allied Health professionals who you can align with and learn and grow from. One such fantastic program is the Business Accelerator Program run by the

Global Kaizen Group where dozens of industry-leading Exercise Physiologists and Allied Health professionals team up on individual and group mentoring sessions, sharing success stories and learnings as well as being guided by systems and templates to implement into their businesses. This type of program also enables face to face conference alignment collaboration on a quarterly basis and with external business professionals who are brought in to enable future growth. It is this type of ongoing professional development that is an absolute must for any budding entrepreneur or small business operator within the Allied Health industry.

Early on in my career I learnt the hard way regarding my education and I only wish I had started this at a younger age. I still remember a mentor of mine saying to me, "Jason, you can only ever grow to your own personal level of incompetence," This one comment alone has driven me to continually improve myself personally and professionally and if you're wanting to see rapid growth and success in your Allied Health company, then it's essential you look to grow and develop in collaboration with industry leaders, those on the same journey as yourself and strong mentors with proven track records in the industry.

Chapter 4:

Niche / USP

We've all heard the comments and instructions over the years to be different to have a unique point of difference that makes you stand out from your competition but rarely in the Allied Health industry do we actually ever see it. For most providers the idea of carving out their own niche or point of difference is exactly that, an idea and not something that they actively work on. Yet it is one of the most powerful tools in your arsenal when starting your Allied Health company or working with a company that's ready to really grow and explode into the market.

Regardless of which way you term it, a niche, USP (unique selling proposition) or point of difference, ultimately it's about having something that is actually worthwhile and valued by prospective clients. It is something that must be leveraged off within the business at every opportunity and formulates the basis for the most successful sales and marketing strategies.

Simply put, a USP is that unique aspect to your company that is going to be much more sought after than the standard operations from your competitors. Is it that you are going to brand your clinic The Knee Clinic to show your unique occupation to working with knees? Your uniqueness may also be based around a service or product that is unique to yourself and your company and not readily available anywhere else. There is also a distinct possibility that your own diversity could almost be its own specialty that you are able to drive your niche from.

Often USP's can be very simple to develop within a company but they're also multilayered and will potentially change in time as the understanding and depth you are able to create will actually fuel a better long-term marketing strategy anyway. Having a strong USP also leads heavily to the development of guarantees and risk reversal strategies which are absolutely essential for people to ultimately buy your product or service. These guarantees are often very simple statements, whether it be a money back guarantee or even just a communication call back guarantee within a particular time frame. Regardless of how small and trivial it may seem, it is these simple-to-manage guarantees that will enable you to remove a client's resistance to buy from you. Keep in mind that you are in the business of health and you must continue to understand that people ultimately are buying your service and hence, having these risk-reversal and minimisation strategies as guarantees within your company, is one of the most effective ways to ensure the closing of more sales and the ability to get more new patients in the door.

We often do large amounts of work with Allied Health practitioners and their teams to better develop not only their niche and unique selling propositions but to also ensure they develop an appropriate strategy to leverage their marketing and sales growth from. It's all good and well to have. Words on a page that you can claim are your points of difference but the next step is to always ensure that it is not only clearly referenced but also followed with a clear strategy of implementation for the marketplace.

The biggest problem that I see within the Allied Health industry is that too many practitioners try to leverage and differentiate themselves by their expertise as a technician. Simply put, you can continually tell people how much better you are or that you have the extra knowledge but in the real world, within the business of health, people are not buying the additional letters after your name or the fact that you have spent more time studying at a university. They are actually going to be sold more easily and much more frequently on the aforementioned unique selling proposition and guarantees that you have in place.

I would strongly encourage all Allied Health practitioners to not create their niche based on what is perceived within our industry as being a niche or benefit but rather what is actually going to be seen by the marketplace as more benefit to them. I'm certainly not detracting from those who do high level studies such as the completing of a PhD but using this high level education as a way to promote your services as being more valued in the private business sector is never going to work. It is those who can display a niche which better risk-minimises their purchasing decision and better assists them to understand the solution you are going to provide them with who will always gain better traction in the marketplace and ultimately gain you more referrals and patients to grow with.

As we are all aware, there is still a majority of the public as well as a large number of doctors and other health professionals who still don't accurately know and understand exactly what some Allied Health professionals such as Exercise Physiologists actually do or can complete. So having a strategy that tries to simply slightly educate them but yet ideally leverages off an apparent high level of understanding of this industry to people who don't understand it in the first place is a recipe for a very non-successful strategy. Hence, I again encourage you to look outside the realms of what your technical ability may be and look to create a point of difference for the marketplace that is going to be perceived and more sought after by the people you are actually wanting to be involved with your business.

It is often the collaboration with other like-minded Allied Health professionals that sees us come up with some of the best points of differences and unique selling propositions for Allied Health companies as it allows a collaborative approach and moves away from the temptation to simply base a niche on a level of understanding that you may have.

I always like to think about Seth Godin's analogy of the purple cow. If you're driving along the road and there's paddock of black and white cows next to you then most of us barely even notice but if we were to see a bright purple cow amongst the black and white cows, then no doubt it would stand out very distinctly and would force us to take note. Most of us would no doubt pull over to the side of the road to have a closer look, ask questions if we were able to and definitely take pictures and post on social media avenues. All of the things that are going to get further attention and eyes on that purple cow. So how are you making your business be the purple cow in the field of black and white cows?

Chapter 5:

Systems

The idea behind having systems in a business and the thoughts that go through most of our heads when we think about a fully systemised business is one of perceived boredom and a task that seems not only too large but one that is definitely not fun in the creation. And for the most part this is true but unless you're wanting to have your business flounder you have absolutely no choice but to work more efficient and effective systems into your business.

When most people in the Allied Health industry think of systems, they would talk about the way a patient is taken from the waiting room into the consultation and back out again after it is all completed. The reality is there is much more to this and the systemisation of your business is not only crucial for long-term success but it is an ever-changing system that will need to be regularly updated. I firmly believe that one of the problems with why people don't introduce systems at the very start of their business is because for most people we are unaware of how to write a system or more specifically we have a generic perception of what a system looks like but unfortunately the difference between this perception and the most effective way of actually completing it is normally miles apart.

For many years now I have been utilising a system-designing process that I have learnt called the 1/10/5 system. This 1/10/5 system is a very simple approach that allows anyone whether it is the business owner or a junior office assistant working on their second day within the team, to easily follow a stepped-out simple process for the completion of any type of system. This is a system that I have learnt and utilised very successfully and have even developed my own template that can simply be printed out and utilised to write in each step. Contrary to what most people believe this system, doesn't actually involve writing step 1 and then step 2 and so on. It actually involves as the title implies, writing step 1 then step 10 then going back to step 5 and continuing through the 1/10/5 system for the completion of a successful system.

This method is the simplest and is also the most effective way. It is basically foolproof and in many respects, makes the writing of systems quite fun. It also means that a large slab of the business can be broken down into many 1/10/5 systems and hence, one or two new systems can be written each and every day so that within several months a fully systemised business will have been completed.

Utilising the default diary I touched on in the earlier chapters, allows the scheduling of a section at the end of each day for the completion of even just one new 1/10/5 system. This will mean that your business is constantly fine tuning and systemising itself over several months and this is a very quick and easy way each day of progressing your business forward. I can also reference learnings from the book *The Slight Edge* that I spoke about before as a further way to ensure your self-discipline in completing these simple, quick and easy daily disciplines to achieve full systemisation will occur in a very short period of time.

Ultimately, all businesses need to be fully systemised so that anyone at any time, is able to complete a particular task. This is none so more evident than when an Allied Health practitioner decides to employ a new team member for the first time. Up until that point the business is the sole practitioner and although many of us want to think that we are irreplaceable, the reality is that often the best thing we can do for our business growth is to actually step aside and allow someone else to complete many of the jobs that we are currently completing. For this to happen successfully, there must be complete systems documented and yes, that will mean there needs to be policies and procedures manuals in place for people to learn from.

1/10/5 System Outline

Overview:
When we have clarity about 'why' this process is needed and how it will help everyone involved, we stand a much greater chance of success in getting the process adopted by our team. Be clear and concise about why this process needs to exist and explain the benefits as well.

The Challenge needing to be systemised: _____

_____

Step 1   1. What would be the 'perfect' first step in this process? When it's done well, what would it look like?
          2.

          3

          4

Step 3   5. Ironically enough, the midway point from start to finish. Defining this allows the team member to stay on track and on time.
          6

          7

          8

          9

Step 2   10. The end! When the process has been executed perfectly, what is the final step and what does it look like?

The best thing about having the 1/10/5 structures and systems in place in document form is that if anything needs to be changed or improved upon, anyone within the organisation can simply pull out that one system and make a minor change to just one or two of the steps before having it inserted back into the document and fully functional again. This is a much more effective use of time, money and energy compared with the standard procedures manuals large companies actually create which for the most part become a useless dormant document that sits on a shelf gathering dust.

Utilising this structure of systemisation that we have developed, you can move forward into much more effective uses of systems including the visual display and learning of systems. With the modern capabilities of our phones we are all able to at any time utilise our camera phones to record a small one-minute video of particular systems which will be better understood than a written version. For those that have their own clinics and team members it is often the small attention to details that become the most frustrating. For example, there's often a particular way you may like a room to be presented or a particular way you like a room to be cleaned and rather than trying to put this into words, it is much easier, quicker and more effective to simply record for one minute the process of exactly how you're wanting the task to be completed. Anyone is then able to watch that small snippet and complete it exactly as they saw it and hence, having videoed systems is a much more effective way of ensuring overall systemisation of your business.

The next major benefit of getting multiple systems involved with your business is the fact that within a short period of time, as your business grows, you will need to be seeking to leverage greater amounts of your time for the completion of tasks by other people or even more so by the use of technology and computerised systems. This avenue of automation and ideal effectiveness can only come about if you have strong and robust systems in places. It is this automation of systems that will greatly see massive growth come at a much more rapid rate for yourself and your business. But it all starts with the completion of these simple daily habits of completing one or two 1/10/5 systems and the piecing together of this from day one. I strongly encourage everyone to work on this each and every day as it is something that takes the smallest amount of time but ensures that your business runs at the most effective rate possible and ultimately frees up more of your time to do more of the essential and important tasks such as obtaining more referrals, enabling growth of the company or seeing additional patients that will only enable the business to obtain more revenue and growth.

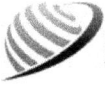

Manage People

How to Manage Induction – First Day

How to Manage Induction- First Day

TM = Team Member

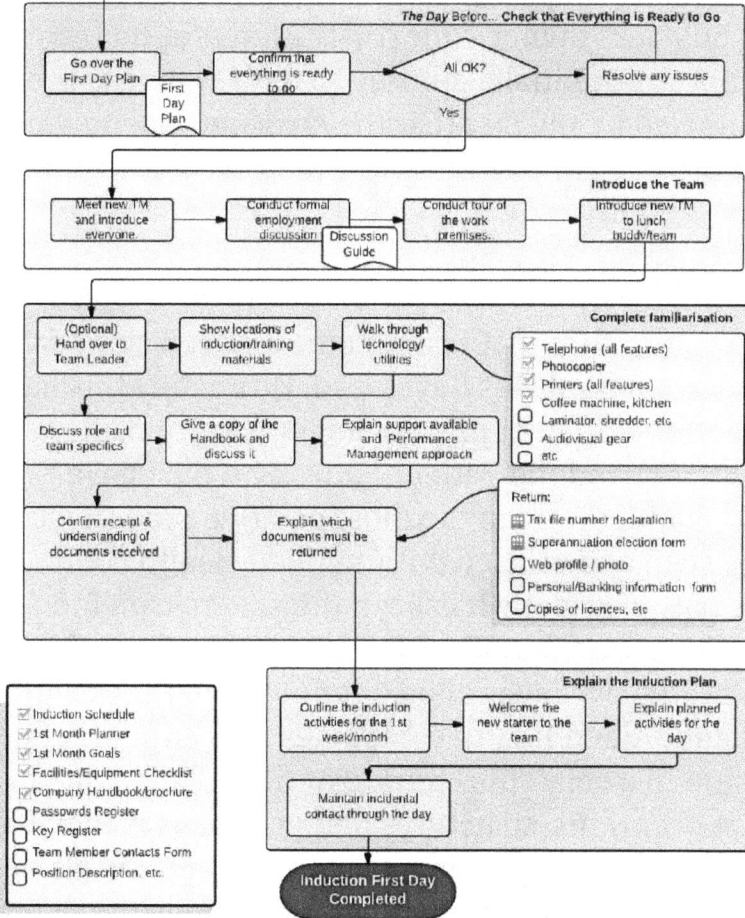

The Day Before... Check that Everything is Ready to Go

- Go over the First Day Plan
- First Day Plan
- Confirm that everything is ready to go
- All OK?
- Yes
- Resolve any issues

Introduce the Team

- Meet new TM and introduce everyone.
- Conduct formal employment discussion
- Discussion Guide
- Conduct tour of the work premises.
- Introduce new TM to lunch buddy/team

Complete familiarisation

- (Optional) Hand over to Team Leader
- Show locations of induction/training materials
- Walk through technology/ utilities

- ☑ Telephone (all features)
- ☑ Photocopier
- ☑ Printers (all features)
- ☑ Coffee machine, kitchen
- ☐ Laminator, shredder, etc
- ☐ Audiovisual gear
- ☐ etc.

- Discuss role and team specifics
- Give a copy of the Handbook and discuss it
- Explain support available and Performance Management approach

Return:
- ▦ Tax file number declaration
- ▦ Superannuation election form
- ☐ Web profile / photo
- ☐ Personal/Banking information form
- ☐ Copies of licences, etc

- Confirm receipt & understanding of documents received
- Explain which documents must be returned

Explain the Induction Plan

- ☑ Induction Schedule
- ☑ 1st Month Planner
- ☑ 1st Month Goals
- ☑ Facilities/Equipment Checklist
- ☑ Company Handbook/brochure
- ☐ Passwords Register
- ☐ Key Register
- ☐ Team Member Contacts Form
- ☐ Position Description, etc.

- Outline the induction activities for the 1st week/month
- Welcome the new starter to the team
- Explain planned activities for the day

- Maintain incidental contact through the day

Induction First Day Completed

Ultimately, in the Allied Health industry, I found the developing of visual flowcharts to be the best way to represent these 1/10/5 systems and these are very easy for anyone to understand. They involve colour and with flowcharts it is almost impossible to get them wrong. This further empowers team members and ensures that as a business owner your frustration around team members potentially getting systems wrong is greatly minimised by the fact that they can't go wrong due to the absolute simplicity of how they are put together and represented.

This mentality towards systemisation and the easy-to-follow structure that I complete, has seen some fantastic systems and policies developed. Ultimately this has led to the development of a Customer Experience Parthenon and the Patient Pathway which have singlehandedly been the most positive growth factor I have seen and utilised within Allied Health companies. This pathway alone has been the sole reason for massive growth in Allied Health companies and it is also something we have rolled out dozens of times within stagnant Allied Health companies to see them turn around in a very short period of time. The reality around these programs, structures and pathways is that although they may seem complicated and are all individualised to each business, the simplicity of them is still based around the initial concepts spoken about earlier in this chapter. These pathways are also something that the members of our Kaizen tribe talk about as being some of the best avenues of growth they have completed in their business.

Regardless of what level you are at with systems in your business, I would strongly encourage you to utilise these simple strategies briefly mentioned above. These systems will provide a more efficient and effective way of stepping out your business and further systemization and automation will occur. You will then be able to find greater ability to work with more patients, see your business grow and ultimately ensure you continually step closer to achieving your long term vision and goals.

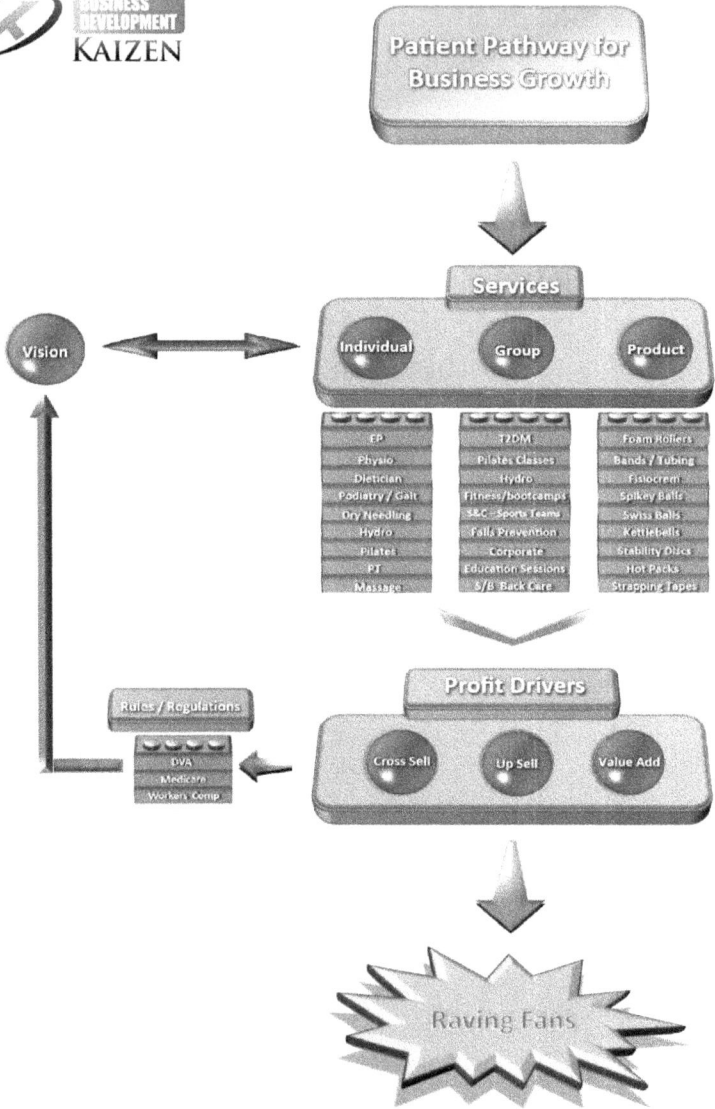

Patient Pathway for Business Growth

KAIZEN — BUSINESS DEVELOPMENT

Vision

Services
- Individual
- Group
- Product

Individual	Group	Product
EP	T2DM	Foam Rollers
Physio	Pilates Classes	Bands / Tubing
Dietician	Hydro	Fisiocrem
Podiatry / Gait	Fitness/bootcamps	Spikey Balls
Dry Needling	S&C - Sports Teams	Swiss Balls
Hydro	Falls Prevention	Kettlebells
Pilates	Corporate	Stability Discs
PT	Education Sessions	Hot Packs
Massage	B/B Back Care	Strapping Tapes

Profit Drivers
- Cross Sell
- Up Sell
- Value Add

Rules / Regulations
- DVA
- Medicare
- Workers Comp

Raving Fans

44

Chapter 6:

Test and Measure

One of the biggest mistakes made by Allied Health practitioners in the health industry is the complete lack of testing and measuring strategies and understanding the numbers and data that are crucial to the survival and more so the improvement and growth of the company.

For the most part all we hear about within the industry is the need to understand your business financials and metrics. Funnily enough this normally comes about from the presentation we have all seen at various times conducted at a seminar or conference by an accountant. There is certainly nothing wrong with this but the truth of the matter stands in the fact that having a profit and loss and balance sheet amongst other reports, done reactively by your accountant every three months at BAS time, is not what your business most needs. In nearly every case of more than 200 Allied Health businesses I have worked with, at some point in time and unfortunately still for many of them, the understanding around what they should be keeping an eye on is formulated from these generalised comments they have received previously regarding their financial markers. Although I'm a very strong supporter of having bookkeepers and accountants as part of your external team, I'm also acutely aware that in the vast majority of situations the data and financial metrics they will provide you with in their reports are retrospective of what has already occurred and unfortunately there is very little, if anything, you can actually do to make changes to the numbers on those reports. Yes, these are better than not having any reports and yes, it does allow you to proactively make changes to improve on your financial situation but the tried and tested proven way is to more effectively test and measure market points before they occur to ensure that you can make the most accurate and beneficial decisions that are going to give you the greatest overall result. By utilising this proactive approach through the test and measure strategies, systems and templates I have designed you are enabled to basically generate these reports that your accountants currently give you several months in advance. It is obviously much more beneficial to know where the business is directly going to be in three, six or twelve months' time than simply being told at tax time that this is what has previously occurred. It allows for a much greater empowerment of yourself personally and professionally and ensures that as the business owner, whether it is you as a sole trader or managing teams with dozens of employees, you are much better equipped to ensure you're making decisions in the best interest of everyone and not just hoping what you are doing is correct while later finding that these decisions could, or should, have been made differently to invoke a more positive result.

A simple statement we have all heard many times no doubt is, "What you can measure, you can manage." Unfortunately most people basically pay lip service to this comment. It is something that all Allied Health businesses should improve on.

The test and measure process can start from the simplest of ideals such as measuring when inquiries are taken and what the conversion rate onto new appointments is. It can be as simple as having a post-it note sitting next to the phone and every time someone calls in to talk about your business, services or have a general inquiry about programs and prices, etc., you are able to record in the first column that an inquiry was made and if you are successful in obtaining an appointment, then you can simply put a mark in the second column signifying a conversion of sale. This is the easiest and most basic form of test and measure and it starts to enable you to gather data on how successful you are at securing the leads in the first place.

This simple strategy can be increased to a one-page table that might include what the topic of inquiry was about, who the referring doctor or health professional was or even looking at what day and time the inquiry came in. These very simple metrics enable you to forecast when the busiest times are for inquiries and the securing of new appointments which ultimately is the growth for your company. It also enables you to coordinate when the best time is to have staff on reception if you are in the early stages of business and only have casual or part-time reception team members. There is also an ability to better understand your sales process and the actual words you use to secure the sale, and for the larger teams, it enables you to better understand and improve particular team members who may not be as successful in securing these inquiries. Although this may all seem very simplistic and have no significant value to your current situation, I would actually challenge this ideal and provide you with evidence that on average the completing of a simple test and measure strategy such as this within the dozens of Allied Health businesses we work within has actually shown to generate on average more than $12,000 of increased revenue with my personal record being a $74,000 yearly revue increase.

I have placed a simple and standardised daily testing and measuring sheet within this chapter and you can see that from a simple table such as this a significant amount of data can easily be tracked and can inform business decisions.

		Repeat Customer		New Customer			Sales Conversion		
Inquiry #	Prospects Name	New Inquiry	Same Inquiry	How Did They Hear About You	Which Marketing Strategy	Details Captured Y/N	Sale Made	Sale Value	Follow Up/Call Back
1									
2									
3									
4									
5									
6									
7									
8									
9									
10									
TOTALS									

Daily Testing and Measuring Sheet

Company: _____   Date: _____

Often, the main challenge behind test and measuring within a business comes down to the business owner's mentality of not quite understanding how easy it can actually occur. In previous chapters I spoke about the systemisation and ultimately the automation of these systems and none are more highly leveraged and automated than the test and measure process within a business. It is exceptionally easy to utilise basic programs such as CRM's or other practice management software to generate this data with a click of a button. There are also dozens of tables and spreadsheets I have developed in programs like Excel that can simply have several numbers from these automated practice management programs entered into the Excel table which then automatically drive forward the proven outcomes to show what a particular strategy is going to complete. These tables are used constantly, time and time again, with stealth accuracy and enable me to ensure that strategies regarding particular programs or marketing that I'm about to engage within can have the outcome predicted before the strategy is even run. Therefore, more successful marketing campaigns are secured time after time which ultimately lead to exponential growth of the Allied Health company with the least amount of risk of the strategy not working. These tables and formulas have been developed over many years of testing and measuring and massive amounts of data across so many businesses and has now become an automated process enabling strong and positive business decisions to be made in a very short period of time with high confidence for the most guaranteed positive outcome.

Behind the test and measure of an Allied Health practice comes simple tables that I have learnt over the years. One of these tables is known as the 5 Ways table which was designed by a friend and mentor of mine, Brad Sugars. By measuring five key markers and understanding how simply they can be applied, all the probability and guesswork about the future numbers of your business can be removed. I have included a copy of this 5 Ways data table for you to start working with but it is just the tip of the iceberg of the benefit your business can see from using these types of test and measure strategies.

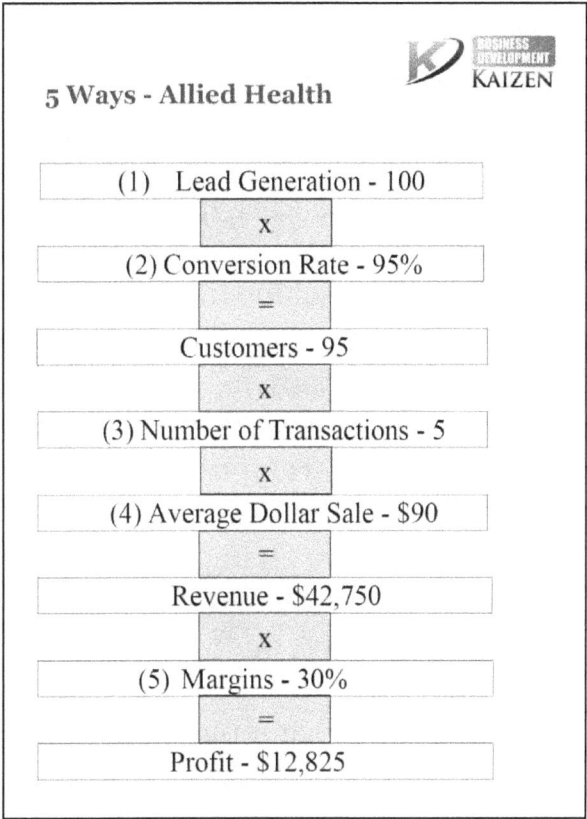

5 Ways - Allied Health   KAIZEN

(1) Lead Generation - 100

X

(2) Conversion Rate - 95%

=

Customers - 95

X

(3) Number of Transactions - 5

X

(4) Average Dollar Sale - $90

=

Revenue - $42,750

X

(5) Margins - 30%

=

Profit - $12,825

If you require further information about the 5 Ways and how to take the next steps in the guaranteed business growth of your company, then feel free to visit the Global Kaizen Group website where we are able to provide you with loads more helpful information and give you the solution you are after.

Once you have the basics down regarding the test and measure side, you are able to further develop these strategies into the completion of utilisation charts for team members. These charts instantly and accurately give the business owner an understanding of work percentages by all team members and where the allocation of time and money within the business is actually being spent. These are further data metrics that few Allied Health businesses currently complete but are absolutely essential to making informed business decisions regarding the expenditure seen within your company, and more so, knowing the perfect time to recruit new team members and grow your business to the next level. Without this type of data being generated you are simply flying blind, without a map, and although you may believe you have an understanding of where your business lies, the truth of the matter is that without the exact numbers in black and white print in front of you, you are simply relying on educated guesswork when making very significant business decisions.

Although the 5 Ways is a good starting point, it is very generic and limiting in nature. You can't cling to the 5 Ways as the best way and only way to do numbers in your Allied Health business.

Allied Health businesses need more specific data than generic test and measure 5 Ways data. It is for this reason that I realised to be a true master of my own Allied Health businesses, I have to master financials specific to Allied Health. It is after many years of fine tuning my own financial mastery that I came up with the Financial Mastery Formula™ specific to the Allied Health industry.

The Financial Mastery Formula™ enables everything proactive that you need to understand the financials currently in your business and what you are needing in the future. It is exceptionally simple and is made up of the only eight numbers you need in your Allied Health business to take full financial control.

I have included an outline of the eight-stack of the Financial Mastery Formula™. It clearly shows how multiple blocks are plugged together to clearly and concisely show everything from sales and marketing through to revenue streams and simple cash flow forecast. It also has avenues to accurately predict team performance based around spec ratings and utilisation of team members. This is the only true way to measure effectiveness and efficiency in Allied Health businesses.

I strongly recommend that anyone running an Allied Health business learns and utilises the Financial Mastery Formula™ as it is the only Allied Health-specific financial formula that enables full retrospective analysis across all avenues of your business and more importantly, proactively enables you to predict and understand exactly where your business numbers will lead you in the coming weeks and months. This is critical to understanding how and when to take on your next team members, open another clinic, how much you can invest in marketing strategies and all other activities in your business.

The test and measure within a business can be used in many different avenues and it is something that is actually quite fun to complete. I utilise tables and structures to automate customer surveys which gives me generated data to track and improve areas of the business based on our patients experience. It also enables us to ensure we are in constant alignment with our vision and alerts us if we need to make changes to our marketing strategies, patient guarantees or much more.

Break-even Analysis – Marketing Campaign

Total Fixed Costs (Ad placement, production)	$...............
Total Variable Costs... (Telephone, wages, rent, etc.)	$...............
Total Delivery Cost... (Taxes, transport, packaging, etc.)	$...............
Total Costs...	$...............
Average $ Sale...	$...............

Total Cost $............... / Average $ Sale...............

=Clients Needed to Break Even: ....

Financial Mastery Formula™

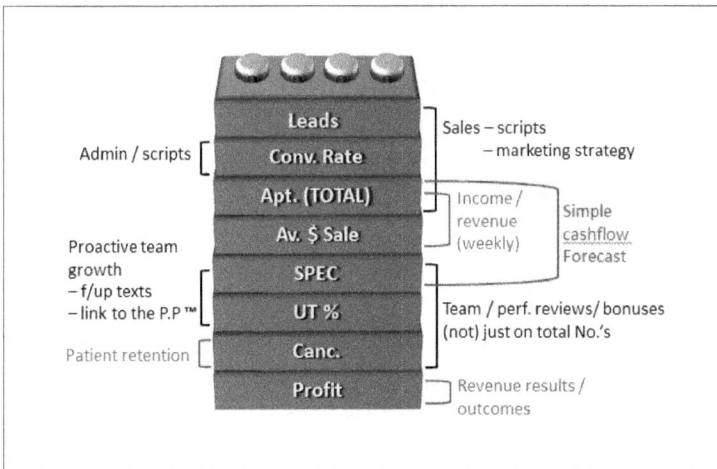

I strongly support every Allied Health practitioner to have a firm understanding of the numbers in their business. This includes having bookkeepers and accountants there to better manage and advise your tax management strategies and future planning. However, in all aspects of business and certainly in our Allied Health field, the real benefit of knowing your numbers doesn't come from these reactive reports but more so from the ability to test and measure and accurately forecast with the simple systems and templates I have discussed. These will ensure you make the most beneficial decisions and have the knowledge and understanding of what the upcoming weeks and months are going to produce in your business. You will be empowered immensely to make more educated business decisions. Knowing this cash flow forecast enables your planning process for business growth regarding recruitment, team growth, technology leverage, equipment and many more business avenues to be decided upon with strong confidence and great accuracy, guaranteeing the best strategy for growth and the sustainability of your business.

Chapter 7:

Developing your team and the culture within

Once all of the previous steps have been completed or have at least been initiated and are being worked upon, the greatest form of leverage to be seen within a company can be addressed. The development of the team which secures the future growth and stability of your Allied Health company.

All businesses must have a strong team and team culture. This is exceptionally evident within the Allied Health industry.

For myself and many of my successful business colleagues in other industries, we always work off the ideal that you "hire on attitude and train on skill". Obviously within Allied Health if you are hiring practitioners, then you are needing to ensure they have the appropriate professional degree and appropriate accreditations behind them before being able to ask them to complete the role. Assuming they have that ability, then it is more imperative to look for someone with the right attitude and consider who is going to be the best team fit rather than simply going for someone who may have done further post graduate studies. I'm certainly not turning people away or encouraging people not to complete further studies and specialisations, but keep in mind that in the Allied Health industry, having the extra letters after your name does not actually give you a greater opportunity at job prospects in the private practice realm of the industry.

When comparing two or three similar potential team members, it is always going to be the team member who is the best team fit for where the company is going that will secure the job and even if the skill level may not be quite the level of others they are competing with for that position, it is actually very easy to provide additional education and training through a variety of means and upskill them where needed. However, trying to change their behavioural and personality traits and hope that they fit into the team will not happen. Hiring just on skill and not on the best team fit always works out to the long term detriment of the company and for many business owners in the early startup phase, it is the worst thing for a company to actually experience.

A strong team must have a strong team culture and after working through the vision and mission of the business developing the *points of culture* of the team are crucial.

Points of Culture ensure that everyone understands the rules of the game. Quite simply put, when playing a game of soccer everyone is aware that when the ball goes out of play, the opposing team will stand on the sideline and throw the ball back in to play before the game recommences. Obviously there are more details and specificity around the exact rule but having all the participants understanding the rules of the game they are all playing is crucial to ensuring the game flows with the minimal amount of disruption. This is exactly the same in all teams. Having everyone within the game knowing what is accepted and what isn't accepted, what can and should be done, ensures the smoothest ability for the business to be effective in achieving its goals.

The points of culture within the team are absolutely essential and it is a process we go through with many teams to help ensure all team members are part of this development process. The points of culture are the fundamental ideals that the team is based upon. They include a statement surrounding each culture point highlighting how the team define the point. This is a very powerful step in ensuring everyone is on the same page and in alignment. It is also the start of a successful recruiting strategy which will see the people most aligned with your team and the journey that your business is actually on, being drawn to your team and making the recruiting and growth phase of your business much easier, smoother and ultimately more successful. You can see more details about the Global Kaizen Group's Points of Culture on the *About Us* page of our website www.globalkaizengroup.com.au.

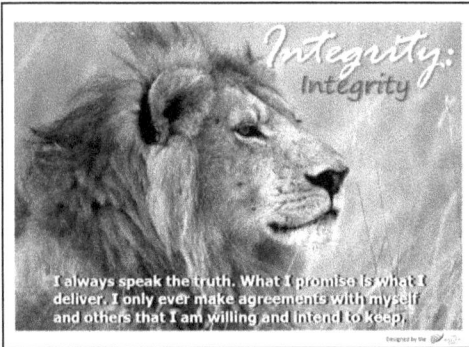

Integrity

I always speak the truth. What I promise is what I deliver. I only ever make agreements with myself and others that I am willing and intend to keep.

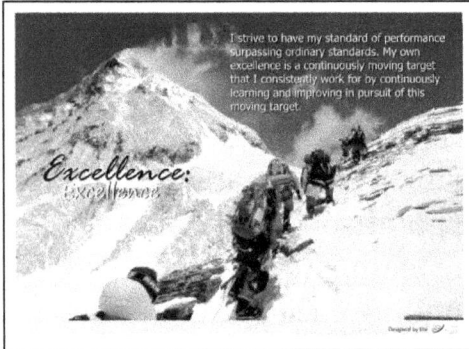

Reciprocity

I believe in always responding in a positive and rewarding manner. I encourage others with kind and friendly actions and greatly aim towards continually giving to others. The showing of gratitude is held very close to me but it does not limit my future growth.

Always grateful, never satisfied.

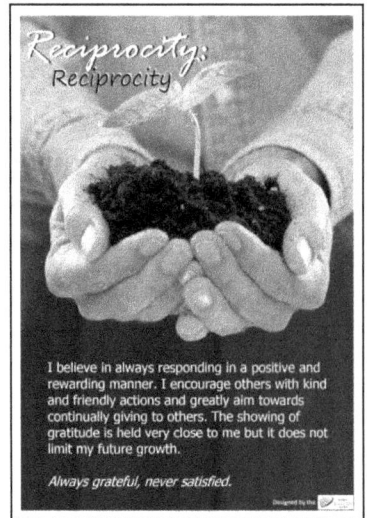

Excellence

I strive to have my standard of performance surpassing ordinary standards. My own excellence is a continuously moving target that I consistently work for by continuously learning and improving in pursuit of this moving target.

The Allied Health industry is predominately made up of professional who are educated to have a thirst for more knowledge, to become better, continually learn and know more than we did yesterday. Although this is very positive it also creates a major challenge to develop over time where a large number of Allied Health professionals have the mentality that they are the best person and that no one else can do the job that they are doing. I see this in all areas of Allied Health and it only helps to fuel a greater competitive drive between colleagues who ultimately should be collaborating more rather than competing. There is a huge amount of work in our industry and I believe that the mentality of always believing you are better than your competitors is often a hampering factor to your business growth and the growth of the industry as a whole.

I'm a firm believer in "coopertition" which is where you are actually in a cooperative relationship with your competitors. In this environment it is a collaboration of growth between everyone that actually enables the industry pie to grow as a whole which is better for everyone's business as opposed to simply trying to singlehandedly grow your slice of the pie to the detriment of your competitors. It is always better to grow the industry pie and see everyone grow than to simply focus on yourself and increase your own slice.

YOU ARE ALLOWED TO ⬇

MAKE
THE DECISION
you think is the right decision to make.

START
SOMETHING
that needs to be started.

ASK
FOR HELP
whenever you want it.

HELP
OTHERS
whenever you can
(even if they don't ask for it).

Don't think for a minute that you're the best at everything in your business. This is a lesson that I learnt the hard way many years ago. Understanding that there is always someone who can do a particular task better than you is the first step to truly seeing your business grow. So focus on what you are great at and concentrate your efforts in that area and be prepared to hire the best and leverage the rest.

Within the Allied Health industry I see so many teams with business owners who want to lead as it is something that is so widely talked about in the last 10 years of business. Leading is obviously very powerful and the ideal goal but so many Allied Health practitioners don't master the step before that which pertains to the management side of working with team members. I would strongly encourage you to read the book *One Minute Manager.* It's a very quick and easy read but in my opinion, it is the best business management book ever written and will empower you to understand the best ways to effectively manage team members.

A leader and leading are not the same thing. Often you can become a leader simply by luck, fortune or even internal politics. However, when you are leading, you must have followers because they are wanting to follow you.

Great leaders inspire others to act through a sense of belonging. There are only two ways to influence human behaviour – through either manipulation or inspiration. When a leader uses manipulation to influence human behaviour, it only leads to transactions occurring and not loyalty. Rather, when a great leader inspires actions it not only leads to an increase in transactions but it also builds lifetime loyalty.

As the leader, manager or owner of the business it is ultimately your responsibility to be the keeper and supporter of the team culture. Even having the mentality of trying to catch someone doing the right thing is a very simple and positive strategy that always adds value to your team. It changes people's mentalities and further leads onto gratitude, reciprocity and a more supportive, cohesive culture that all teams must embrace in order to be on a stable and continued path to growth.

Recently, I was very privileged to be one of a very select few to spend a day with Seth Godin on the only day he spent with people on his first ever trip to Australia. Although this was a fantastic day with some amazing learnings and gold nuggets from one of the world's best, probably the best lesson I learned on that day was his phrase, "People like us, do things like this." It is something that I have held with me and rolled out in several of my companies and also encourage the dozens of Allied Health practitioners in our Kaizen tribe to embrace. This mentality ensures a leadership focus of setting the bar and making everyone within the team realise that what you're doing is not actually anything that amazing. It is simply what we are all meant to be doing at all times because "people like us do things like this". I encourage you to work with this mantra yourself and with your own teams and watch the power of this principle unfold.

The holding of team days and festivities for team members is an absolutely crucial step for your business to grow. Even if you only have a business with one other person, then you should make a regular habit to take that person out to lunch or engage in non-work, fun-based activities because "the teams that play together, stay together". The minimal amount of money you spend on your team you will soon understand to be the best form of return on investment a business owner can ever make.

Understanding that your team, and the culture to which your team is aligned, will be your biggest asset for future business growth. Knowing that a strong team will crawl over broken glass to help the team push forward is one of the most exciting things to see as a business owner. Keep in mind that the team you have, or the team you are planning on having, will be your business' best asset for growth and it all starts with the culture you develop and foster along the journey.

Chapter 8:

Conclusion

The setting up of a highly successful Allied Health clinic is one that takes the patience and dedication of the business owner and the team. Ultimately, there are these 7 fundamentals, imperative for the business owner to get operating at the earliest possible time. Once these 7 fundamentals are initiated it does take an ongoing commitment to go into much greater detail and ensure that the specific details and in-depth areas within these key fields are explored, designed and implemented.

This book, does not address many other areas of great importance to an Allied Health clinic such as the specific marketing and promotion and the sales strategies behind the selling of your health business. These areas are much more complex than simply writing a few pages in a book. They are areas of Allied Health businesses that I am very passionate about and that I provide mentoring and coaching for.

Within the Global Kaizen Group Business Development programs and membership site we offer a extensive advice, systems, templates and case studies highlighting the best strategies on how to market and promote your business.

There are also significant components including the development of technology and people leverage within your company and the formulation of in-depth strategies that will further secure your business success. All of this information, along with the internationally awarded Allied Health Business Blueprint that I have developed are contained within the Global Kaizen Group Business Development Program. This program is something that I am very proud of and has seen exceptional benefit to every Allied Health business owner who has been involved. I truly believe that the way we are providing education to our industry is enabling the whole industry pie to grow together. Collaboratively we are allowing for an improved health business landscape for all of us to grow and thrive within whilst also making the most benefit to the Australian health landscape surrounding us.

If you are wanting more information, systems, templates, checklists, programs, marketing advice, recruitment strategies and anything else that comes with a seven-figure Allied Health company, then please contact our team or get more information at www.globalkaizengroup.com.au. All of our programs come with money back guarantees to ensure that there is no risk for you in securing the Allied Health clinic of your dreams.

The Allied Health industry is something that I am exceptionally passionate about and although there have been many tough times, it is also an industry that has been very kind to myself. I believe that if we all work together, share and collaborate our successful strategies, then as a health industry we will all achieve greater heights of success and enable the overall health landscape of Australia to change.

I'm very grateful for you reading my book and trust that you have received significant benefit. Here's to your lifestyle abundance!

AWARDS

The following is a list of just some of the prestigious awards Jason Pilgrim and his companies have received:

2015 – **Winner** - Business Excellence Award, Pacific Asia Region – Best Marketing Campaign

2015 – **Winner** – ESSA Exercise Physiologist Advocate of the Year

2014 – **Winner** - Business Excellence Award, Pacific Asia Region – Best Service Company

2013 – **Winner** – Business Excellence Awards, Pacific Asia Region – Best Overall Company

2013 - **Finalist**– Business Excellence Awards, Pacific Asia Region – Entrepreneur of the Year

2012 - **Winner** – Business Excellence Awards, Pacific Asia Region – Most Community Impact

2012 – **Winner** - Australian Small Business Awards – Health Improvement Services

2011 – **Winner** – Local Business Awards – Business Person of the Year

2011 - **Winner** – Local Business Awards – Best Professional Services

2011 – **Winner** - International Business Excellence Awards – Most Community Impact

2011 – **International Finalist** – International Business Excellence Awards - Young Entrepreneur of the Year – Jason Pilgrim

2010 – **Winner** – Australian Small Business Young Entrepreneur of the Year

2010 – **National Finalist** – Australian Small Business Awards - Professional Services

2010 – **National Finalist** – Australian Small Business Awards - Rapid and Sustained Growth

2010 – **Finalist** – 2UE Young Gun Award with MyBusiness Awards– Jason Pilgrim

2009 – **National Finalist** – Australian Small Business Awards - Best New Business

2009 – **Winner** - NSW/ACT Best New Small Business

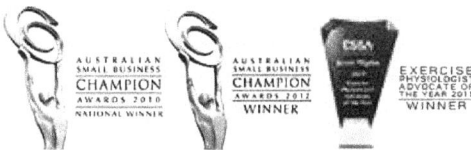

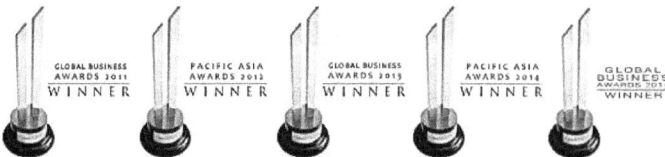

Learn from Australia's most awarded Allied Health Professional

Get instant access to industry-leading templates, systems, cheat sheets, proven strategies and Australia's only internationally awarded Allied Health business blueprint.

Launch Program

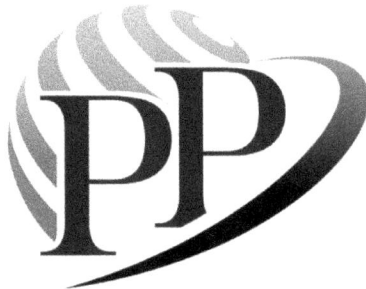

— THE —
Profitable Practice

POWERED BY GLOBAL KAIZEN GROUP

The Global Kaizen Group's **Launch Program** is a two-month business development program specific to Allied Health business owners. There is no other program in the industry like it and it also includes the following internationally awarded signature systems:

- **The GP Signature System™**
- **The Patient Pathway™**
- **The Financial Mastery Formula™**
- **The Allied Health Business Blueprint™**
- **The Patient Referral Maximiser™**
- **The Perfect Recruitment Pipeline™**

The completion of the two-month **Launch Program** gives you access to everything outlined here and also includes attendance at a two-day face-to-face business conference and access to the closed Facebook group with Australia's leading Allied Health providers that share ideas, strategies and success stories.

The Launch Program is a total risk-free opportunity for you to create explosive growth in your practice. This includes a 100% money back guarantee to ensure your future success with this program.

- Do you want more referrals?
- Do you want guaranteed growth for your health business?
- Do you want the proven systems and templates to save you time and money?
- Do you want access to Australia's most awarded Allied Health Business Blueprint?

JOIN THE
KAIZEN TRIBE

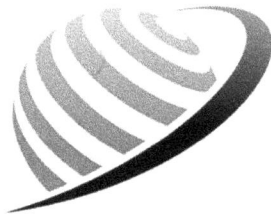

GLOBAL
KAIZEN
GROUP

KAIZEN, THE POWER BEHIND YOUR ALLIED HEALTH PRACTICE

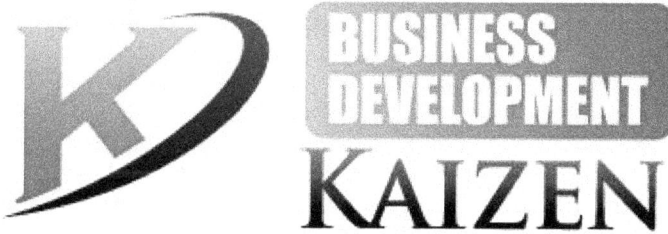

- ➢ Conferences
- ➢ One on one Business Strategy Sessions
- ➢ Membership Site Access
- ➢ Private Facebook Page
- ➢ Networking / Mentoring
- ➢ Accountability Buddy System

www.globalkaizengroup.com.au

www.ingramcontent.com/pod-product-compliance
Lightning Source LLC
Chambersburg PA
CBHW070917280326
41934CB00008B/1754